Food Fit

A NON-DIET APPROACH TO
HEALTHY EATING & WEIGHT LOSS.

Tasha Sarver, RD, LD, CDE

Food Fit: A non-diet approach to healthy eating and weight loss.
©2018 by Tasha Sarver

Published by Food Fit Nutrition, LLC.
PO Box 681564
Franklin, TN 37064
615-656-8114

Printed and bound in the United States of America.

Editing by Kamahria Hopkins

Cover design by Freepik

ISBN: 978-0-692-12784-1

For more information visit:
www.foodfitnutrition.com

Acknowledgements

Dear God, thank you for giving me the vision to write this book.

My husband Chris Sarver: Thank you for always believing in me, sometimes more than I believe in myself. You are one of the best things to ever happen to me and I am a better person because of you. I love you!

My son Jaxon Sarver: You are the greatest gift that God has ever blessed me with. You are my inspiration to be more successful than I ever dreamed. I love you with every part of me.

My dad Stephen Prince: Thank you for teaching me that in life sometimes you fall, but it is okay as long as you don't stay there. You have inspired and motivated me to be better than I ever thought I could be. Thank you for always being there for me.

My mom Angela Mickens: Thank you for instilling self-confidence in me at a very young age. You are the reason I walk with my shoulders back and head high.

My bonus mom Karen Prince: Thank you for always treating me like I was born in your heart.

My siblings Dale, Dominick, Dennis, Jerome, and Brittney: Each of you have supported me in absolutely everything I have attempted in my life. No matter the distance between us, I always feel your love. Love, your Big Sis!

My cousins/best friends Christina & Kendra: You are both my counselors, voices of reason, cheerleaders, and the absolute best support system a girl could ask for. Thank you for always accepting and loving me, flaws and all.

I dedicate this book in honor of my wonderful grandma Gloria (Mickens) Massey. Grandma, you were my favorite person on earth and you have been my favorite angel since 1999. I am eternally grateful for all the lessons you taught me. I am thankful that you showed me the love of God through your actions. Everything I do is to make you proud.

CONTENTS

Medical Disclaimer

The information provided in this book is for general educational purposes only and not a substitute for medical care. Please consult with your health care provider regarding the diagnosis or treatment of any medical condition prior to starting a new eating and exercise regimen.

Each day you will read a new food fit tip. After reading the tip, you will have the opportunity to think about where you are concerning the tip and then write your goals in the journal. At the end of each week, you will have the opportunity to reflect and journal your progress for the week.

Before beginning, I encourage you to complete the Food Fit Tracker. This will give you the opportunity to track your journey along the way. You can track your starting point, 4 weeks post, and 12 weeks post.

Food Fit Tracker

Date:	Start	4 weeks	12 weeks
Height			
Weight			
Waist			
Chest			
Upper thigh			
Buttocks			

My Journey

Twice in my life I have had to intentionally lose weight. After graduating college in my mid-twenties, there was a huge change in my lifestyle. I went from broke college student eating ramen noodles to working woman eating at restaurants a couple times per week. On top of that, I went from exercising at the university gym to no exercise at all. Like many of you, I knew that my lifestyle habits had not changed for the better. I studied Nutrition in college, so I knew all too well what healthy eating and exercise looked like. I told myself that I deserved to eat out as much as I did. Almost two years later, I had gained over 40 pounds. My clothes no longer fit, my thighs rubbed together, and I was no longer physically fit. I was starting my dietetic internship – a step one must complete to become a dietitian. I made my mind up that I did not want to be the unhealthy dietitian that pointed my finger at others, while I too was struggling with unhealthy eating habits and no exercise. It took me about 30 days to change my way of thinking from do what you want, to change your lifestyle.

At the age of 39, I delivered a healthy baby boy via C-section. While I was pregnant with my son, I gained 42 pounds. My doctor suggested weight gain of no more than 35 pounds, so I don't think I did too bad. What I did fail in was eating healthy during my pregnancy. I blame the hormones because while I was pregnant I hated the taste of vegetables and I craved crunchy salty foods. I am a vegetarian, so the fact that I could not stand the taste of vegetables was a big deal for me. I did not exercise at all during my pregnancy. I experienced a miscarriage with my first pregnancy, so I was scared to exercise in fear that I might lose my baby. So, you guessed it, I ate a lot of crunchy, salty, fatty foods and I was a couch potato for 9 months. After the birth of my son, I was so busy being a new mom that I was not initially concerned with losing weight. Everyone tells you the weight will fall off, but they fail to mention that it's because you are too busy or too tired to eat. Well, the weight did not fall off me completely. After losing about 20 pounds without effort, the weight loss stopped. I set a goal for myself to be back to my pre-pregnancy weight by my 40th birthday. Just in case you are the type of person who likes to know the ending of a book or movie right away, I'll let you know that I made it to my 40th birthday only 4 ½ pounds away from my pre-pregnancy weight.

This 30-day journal contains the tips that I have used twice to meet my weight loss goals. These tips are also the same recommendations that I have given clients who have desired weight loss, improved blood sugar control, improved cholesterol levels, or to just live a healthier lifestyle. If you are not currently meeting your health goals, this book will help you get a lot closer to your goals in just 30 days.

Beverages

Growing up as a kid, I was raised on Kool-Aid. And not just the mix, but the too much sugar type of Kool-Aid, so I enjoyed other sweetened beverages too like lemonade and soda. I remember my grandmother was always trying to lose weight, so she would drink diet Coke. Now diet Coke was not my thing, but I knew the key was to stop drinking my calories. I switched to Crystal Light and good ole bottled water. Eventually, I would start to like diet soda, but in my mid-twenties this was not the case.

Food Fit Tips

Choose:

- Water/Low calorie flavored water
- Unsweetened Tea
- Diet Soda
- Sugar-free low-calorie drink mixes

Which high-calorie beverages do you consume?

_____

_____

_____

_____

_____

Which low-calorie beverages are you willing to trade it for?

_____

_____

_____

_____

_____

What are your beverage goals?

_____

_____

_____

_____

_____

Exercise

I know what you are thinking. Why doesn't she just stick with the first behavior change of beverage choice for a while before changing another habit? Well, that may work for some but not me. The more time I take to change, the more excuses I give to delay changes.

I know from my college days that when I exercised I wanted to eat healthier. Plus, it gave me more energy and made me feel good. Who doesn't need more energy? I decided that four times a week, I would walk on the treadmill for 60 minutes. At the time, I lived in an apartment complex with a small fitness center, so it wouldn't cost me any additional money to exercise. Once I began to actively exercise each week, I was invited to participate in an African Aerobics class. This class was held twice a week and lasted 2 hours. This class was free. I changed my exercise routine to treadmill twice a week and African Aerobics class twice a week.

As a working wife and mother, I don't always have time to go to a gym. I have found On-Demand exercise videos via my cable provider to be very helpful in achieving my exercise goals. I can choose the length of the video that fits my schedule and it can all be done in the privacy of my home.

Food Fit Tips

- Exercise most days of the week for 30 – 60 minutes
- Walk/Run in your neighborhood
- Walk at work during your lunch break
- Purchase a gym membership
- Find On-Demand exercise videos via your cable provider
- Mark exercise on your calendar as part of your daily routine
- Be flexible

- Do something you enjoy
- Find a free class to attend in your community

What exercise can you commit to?

_____
_____
_____
_____
_____

How often will you commit to exercise?

_____
_____
_____
_____
_____

What are your barriers to exercise?

_____
_____
_____
_____
_____

How can you overcome your barriers to exercise?

_____

_____

_____

_____

_____

Fast Food

I became a fast food junkie after college. I stopped cooking and purchased all my meals outside of my home. But fast food comes with a price, and I'm not talking dollars. Many fast food items are high fat, high sugar, and high calorie, which are not healthy when consumed as frequently as I did. I had to go back to my upbringing. As a child, my grandmother cooked dinner daily and fast food was a treat every now and then.

Each week I would make a list of what I was going to eat for the week. I used this list for shopping and meal planning. I'm ok with eating leftovers, so I would make 2-3 meals a week and eat leftovers. I saved so much money by eating at home.

If you cannot cook, there are many places that do meal preparation for you. They will deliver the meal to your home and then you prepare the meal following the instructions provided.

Food Fit Tips
- Eat meals prepared at home most days of the week (see my favorite home-cooked meal, p. 15)
- When dining out, choose healthier options
- Grill or bake more often than frying
- Watch your portion sizes
- Order a kid's meal
- Order a single patty burger vs. a double or triple burger
- Order a small/medium fry vs. a large fry

How often do you eat away from home?

_____

_____

_____

_____

_____

How often are your meals high fat and high calories?

_____

_____

_____

_____

_____

How often are you willing to commit to cooking at home?

_____

_____

_____

_____

_____

If you are unable to cook, what resources will you use to eat healthier meals?

_____

_____

_____

_____

_____

My favorite home cooked meal is spaghetti. My mother taught me how to make my own spaghetti sauce. Over the years, I stopped using her recipe and created my own meatless recipe.

Ingredients
- 1 can Tomato Sauce
- 1 can tomato paste
- 1 large green pepper
- 1 yellow onion
- 6 cloves of garlic
- Italian seasoning
- Garlic salt
- Pepper
- Basil leaves
- Parsley Flakes
- Spaghetti Noodles
- Morning Star Grillers Crumbles
- Vegetable oil of your choice

Directions
1. In a large pot, boil water. Cook spaghetti noodles until done and drain water.
2. In a large skillet, heat a small amount of vegetable oil in the skillet and add 1 bag of Morning Star Grillers Crumbles until completely warm.
3. Chop the green pepper, onion, and garlic.
4. Add vegetables to the skillet with the crumbles. Add the Italian seasoning, garlic salt, pepper, basil leaves, and parsley flakes to taste.
5. In a separate pot, add the tomato sauce and tomato paste. For a chunkier sauce, add more tomato paste. Once completely warm, add to crumbles.
6. Add the spaghetti noodles to the meatless sauce.
7. Enjoy!

Is it a craving or an addiction?

According to dictionary.com, a craving is "a great or eager desire; yearning."

According to dictionary .com, an addiction is "the state of being enslaved to a habit or practice or to something that is psychologically or physically habit-forming."

When I was a child, I was a very picky eater. Some adults in my family would bribe me into eating my food by telling me I would get to eat dessert. Eating something sweet each day turned into a habit that I maintained throughout my adult years. Sweets come with an excessive cost, and that cost is high sugar, high fat, and high calories. These three things were hindering me from being a healthy eater and hindering my weight loss. I decided to switch my cakes, cookies, and candy to fruit. Fruit is naturally sweet, but it is low in calories and low fat. Now I still allow myself to consume sweets but not every day. My goal is to consume sweets no more than twice a week.

Food Fit Tips
- Decrease how often you consume the food you crave
- Find healthier alternatives if necessary
- Don't deprive yourself

What food are you addicted to?

_____

_____

_____

_____

_____

How can you decrease how often you consume this food?

_____

_____

_____

_____

_____

List healthier alternatives for this food(s)?

_____

_____

_____

_____

_____

Salt

Are you the type of person that puts salt on your food before even tasting it? Well, that used to be me. Did you know that 1 tsp of salt has more than 2300 mg of sodium? This is a whole day's intake of sodium; however, we forget that sodium is already found in foods. Canned goods, deli meats, cheese, & pre-packaged foods are the most common.

Do you have high blood pressure, kidney disease, or heart disease? If so, I'm certain your physician has already recommended that you consume low sodium foods.

Eating healthy is not just about weight, it is about healthy choices for a healthier you.

Food Fit Tips
- Choose foods with less than 500 mg of sodium per meal
- 150 mg or less is considered a low sodium food
- Season your foods with herbs or other seasonings to add flavor (Bay leaf, black pepper, garlic powder, oregano, parsley, rosemary, sage, thyme)

Do you believe you consume too much salt?

_____

_____

_____

_____

_____

Which foods do you consume that may be high in salt/sodium?

_____

_____

_____

_____

_____

What are you willing to do to decrease your salt/sodium intake?

_____

_____

_____

_____

_____

Day 6

Eat Breakfast

Breakfast is an important meal each day. Let's break down the word breakfast (break-fast). We all fast at night when we sleep. Our metabolism slows down because there is not much work to do when we are not eating. Breakfast literally breaks the fast. Many people who skip breakfast tend to eat more at other meals or throughout the day. Eating regular meals can help decrease how much you're eating because you are no longer waiting until you are starving to eat. More frequent meals may be beneficial to helping your metabolism work more effectively. Think of your metabolism as a fire. Think of the food you eat as wood. If you start a fire in your fireplace and the wood burns out, the fire goes out. If you are not eating food, your metabolism is working less. I strive to eat breakfast within an hour of waking up each day. It doesn't have to be a large meal.

Food Fit Tips
Quick breakfast ideas:
- Fruit with yogurt
- Slice of toast with peanut butter
- Cereal bar
- Crackers with peanut butter or cheese

How many days of the week do you eat breakfast?

_____
_____
_____
_____
_____

What are your barriers to eating breakfast most days of the week?

_____

_____

_____

_____

_____

What are your quick breakfast choices?

_____

_____

_____

_____

_____

Reflection

You have made it through a whole week of tips, so now it is time to reflect.

What habits have you started to change?

_____

_____

_____

_____

_____

What areas can you still improve in?

_____

_____

_____

_____

_____

What are you most proud of this week?

_____

_____

_____

_____

_____

If you struggled in more than 2 areas, plan how you will do better next week.

_____

_____

_____

_____

_____

If you were successful in implementing 3 or more healthy habits this week, pat yourself on the back and keep the momentum going.

"Today is the tomorrow you talked about yesterday." ~Author unknown

Do it Today!

Carbohydrates

Some people feel like the word carbohydrate is a bad word. Many people have told me that they avoid eating carbohydrates to eat healthier. Carbohydrates are not bad. In fact, your body requires carbohydrates as an energy source. It is the main energy source for your brain. The problem is that most people eat way too many carbohydrates since they are unfamiliar with appropriate portions.

Carbohydrates include starches (bread, rice, pasta, cereal), starchy vegetables (corn, peas, potatoes), fruit, fruit juice, milk, yogurt, & sweets/desserts.

Many of the foods we consume are carbohydrates, but some of you have been unaware of the food sources. Lots of carbohydrates contain fiber. High fiber foods make you feel full faster, so you tend to not eat as much. Fiber allows your body to slowly turn the food to glucose to prevent post-meal blood glucose spikes. Carbohydrates provide the body with lots of vitamins and minerals that are necessary for nutritional health.

Food Fit Tips
- Choose complex carbohydrates such as brown rice, wheat bread, whole wheat pasta, beans, potatoes with the skin.
- Eat the skin on your fruit for additional fiber

Did you know that so many food types are carbohydrates?

_____
_____
_____
_____
_____

Do you struggle with eating too many carbohydrates because you are unaware of the appropriate portions sizes?

_____

_____

_____

_____

_____

Name a few complex carbohydrates that you currently enjoy.

_____

_____

_____

_____

_____

Portion Control

While many people are searching for the miracle pill for weight loss the reality is it is all about portion control. We must consume fewer calories than we burn each day to promote weight loss. It really is simple math: there must be a deficit to lose.

Portion control can be achieved in many ways. Being Food Fit means finding what works for you.

1. Plate method. The plate method is easy to incorporate because it simply requires a plate. This method allows you to eat more of the food choices you enjoy; however, your calories are limited. ½ plate non-starchy vegetables, ¼ plate protein, ¼ plate carbohydrates

2. Count calories. A dietitian can calculate approximately how many calories you require to promote weight loss/maintenance. Using food labels and/or measuring food intake each day, you avoid consuming more than the allotted calorie amount per day.

3. Carbohydrate Counting. People who are living with diabetes and/or pre-diabetes count carbohydrates to help control blood glucose levels. This method can also be used for portion control. This method can really be successful for people who know that they eat way too many carbohydrates each day. A dietitian or diabetes educator can calculate the amount of carbohydrates to limit each day along with guidelines for protein and vegetables.

So which method works best? The method that works best is the one that you can follow.

Food Fit Tips
- Ditch the diet mentality.
- Implement a healthy eating pattern that you can follow long-term.
- It is going to take some effort on your part. Put in the work because it is worth it.

Which portion control method(s) have you tried in the past?

_____

_____

_____

_____

_____

If you have tried a portion control method, what worked best about it?

_____

_____

_____

_____

_____

What portion control method do you plan to try on this Food Fit Journey?

_____

_____

_____

_____

_____

Fat

The reason why we like fat is because it makes food taste so good. Growing up I am certain that at least 90% of the foods I was given as a child included some type of fat. My grandmother kept a can of shortening on her stove and it was used to prepare many of the meals we consumed. Most vegetables contained some type of fatty meat that would help the vegetables taste even better.

The biggest muscle in our bodies is our heart. Eating too much fat or foods that contain cholesterol can increase our risk for developing heart disease.

Saturated fats and trans fats are the types of fats that we should limit in our diets. Saturated fats can be found in animal products such as meat, butter, cheese, and milk. Trans fats are man-made fats that can be found in processed foods, fast foods, and pre-packaged foods.

When you decrease the fat content in your meals and snacks it will decrease your calorie content which will be beneficial to your weight loss goals.

Food Fit Tips
- Choose foods low in fat & cholesterol
- Choose meals with < 12 g fat per meal
- Choose snacks with </= 5 g fat per snack

How often do you eat foods that are high in fats?

_____

_____

_____

_____

_____

How can you decrease how often you consume foods high in fat?

_____

_____

_____

_____

_____

When you think of the high fat food choices that you enjoy, are there any healthy alternatives available?

_____

_____

_____

_____

_____

Cholesterol

At this point in my life I have never had high cholesterol; however, being food fit means being conscious about all the things that can decrease my nutritional health. I have worked with clients who were diagnosed with high cholesterol and we were able to quickly decrease their cholesterol with just making dietary changes.

Foods high in cholesterol are also found in animal products such as eggs, meat, poultry, fish, and dairy.

Cholesterol cannot be dissolved in the blood; therefore, it begins to create a waxy substance that can block your arteries and increase your risk of a heart attack or stroke.

Food Fit Tips
- Consume less than 300 mg of cholesterol per day
- Increase your fiber intake to help decrease your cholesterol
- Ask your doctor what your total cholesterol is at your next visit

Do you know what your total cholesterol level is?

_____

_____

_____

_____

_____

How often do you consume foods that are high in cholesterol?

_____

_____

_____

_____

_____

How do you plan to decrease your cholesterol intake?

_____

_____

_____

_____

_____

Day 12

Fiber

The only time most people think about their fiber intake is when they are constipated. This is when you are not able to have a bowel movement on a regular schedule. I admit that growing up I suffered from constipation a lot. Looking back, it is not surprising because I ate very little vegetables or grains. My diet was high in fat and fried potatoes. I've always been a potato foodie.

Fiber is a key component of many different elements of nutritional health. Diets high in fiber can help decrease cholesterol, increase the feeling of fullness (satiety) with meals, help improve constipation, and help delay glucose absorption.

Foods that are high in fiber include whole wheat bread, brown rice, whole wheat pasta, vegetables, the skin of fruit, bran cereal, and beans to name a few.

Food Fit Tips
- Consume 25 – 35 grams of fiber a day
- Choose high fiber foods at each meal or snack to meet your daily needs
- Use a food diary to track how much fiber you are consuming to see if you are meeting your needs

Are you consuming 25 – 35 grams of fiber per day?

_____

_____

_____

_____

_____

If not, what are your plans to incorporate more fiber in your diet?

_____

_____

_____

_____

_____

Protein

Growing up, I was offered protein with at least two meals a day. Oftentimes things become a habit without you even realizing it. As a result of my upbringing, I typically consume protein with all my meals.

When I became a vegetarian over 8 years ago, it became even more important that I focus on consuming enough protein to meet my needs since I do not consume meat of any kind.

Protein is essential for the growth and repair of muscles. Don't forget that the heart is the largest muscle in the body. Protein also provides a feeling of fullness with meals, which helps you feel satisfied longer between meals. If you have diabetes, protein can help delay the absorption of glucose to prevent a blood glucose spike post-meal. When trying to achieve weight loss you are often consuming less food, so your intake of lean protein can assist you with feeling full.

Protein sources include: beef, poultry, fish, seafood, pork, milk, yogurt, beans, tofu, peanut butter, cheese, tempeh, & lentils to name a few.

Food Fit Tips
- Include a protein source with each meal or snack
- Choose lean protein

What protein sources do you frequently consume?

_____

_____

_____

_____

_____

Do you consume protein with each one of your meals? If no, why not?

_____

_____

_____

_____

_____

Reflection

You have made it through a whole week of tips, so now it is time to reflect.

What habits have you started to change?

_____

_____

_____

_____

_____

What areas can you still improve in?

_____

_____

_____

_____

_____

What are you most proud of this week?

_____

_____

_____

_____

_____

If you struggled in more than two areas, plan how you will do better next week.

_____

_____

_____

_____

_____

If you were successful in implementing three or more healthy habits this week, pat yourself on the back and keep the momentum going.

You are not trying to be perfect, you are striving for consistency.

Water

I never enjoyed drinking water until I was in college. As a kid, the only time I would drink water was if I was playing outside during the summer. And I drank from the water hose. My grandma had a "no running in and out of my house" rule, so the water hose was my only option if I wanted to stay outside. I had a cousin whose family would always drink water. It's funny to say now, but back then I thought it was weird that they drank water. I grew up drinking Kool-Aid with lots of sugar or soda. It wasn't until college that I realized that I was not making the best choices for my health or weight. I did not realize how many calories were in Kool-Aid or soda. My grandma drank diet soda but she would never allow me to at that time.

Did you know that half of your body is made up of water? Why do people feel bad when they are dehydrated? It's because the body needs water. If you are trying to achieve weight loss, water is important because it is a zero-calorie beverage.

Food Fit Tips
- Add lemon or cucumbers to water for additional flavor
- Try sparkling water
- Increase your intake of water by keeping water with you for easy access

How many 8oz cups of water do you drink a day?

_____

_____

_____

_____

_____

If you drink less than 6 (8oz) cups of water per day, what can you do to increase your water intake?

_____

_____

_____

_____

_____

Alcohol

I have always considered myself to be a rare occasion type of alcohol drinker. I reserve alcohol intake for special occasions like my birthday. It's not that I don't enjoy adult beverages, but I choose not to waste my calories on beverages. Alcohol can contain a lot of calories, especially when you consider the size and number of drinks one may consume.

Growing up, I had an Aunt who would drink beer every day and she happened to have a beer gut. I've always associated alcohol with big bellies. Just my perspective as a kid. As a dietitian, I have had clients who have successfully lost weight just by decreasing their alcohol intake without making any other significant dietary changes.

Food Fit Tips
- It is recommended that women consume no more than 1 drink a day
- It is recommended that men consume no more than 2 drinks a day

How frequently do you consume alcohol?

_____

_____

_____

_____

_____

Is your alcohol intake hindering you from reaching your food fit goals?

_____

_____

_____

_____

_____

What changes would you like to make in your alcohol intake?

_____

_____

_____

_____

_____

Snacks

Oftentimes when you think of snacks, you may think of junk food (chips, cookies, candy). Although these are types of snacks, snacks can be and often should be comprised of healthy foods.

Have you ever skipped a meal, so right before the next meal you felt like you were starving, which caused you to over eat at that meal? Well of course you have. Most people have.

Avoid going longer than 5 hours between meals by consuming a planned and healthy snack. Planned is the important part so that you don't get stuck with unhealthy choices. You want something to curb your appetite in between meals, while avoiding excessive calorie intake.

Healthy snacks include anything you like that is low fat, low cholesterol, and lower calorie.

Food Fit Tips
Examples of healthy snacks include:
- Fruit (fresh, canned, or dried)
- Nuts (limit to a handful to keep calories low)
- Crackers with peanut butter
- Crackers with cheese
- 6 oz. Low-fat yogurt
- Baby carrots or celery sticks
- Lettuce wrap (lettuce with scoop of tuna or egg salad)

How frequently do you consume snacks each day?

_____

_____

_____

_____

_____

What type of snacks do you frequently consume?

_____

_____

_____

_____

_____

If this is an area that needs improvement, what are some healthy snack alternatives that you can consume?

_____

_____

_____

_____

_____

Vitamin & Minerals

As a young girl, I remember being offered my Flintstone vitamins every day. I was a very picky eater, so my vitamins were very necessary for optimal nutrition, growth, and development.

Vitamins and minerals are found naturally in the fruits and vegetables that you consume. The question is: Do you consume the appropriate amount of fruits and vegetables each day to meet your nutritional needs? The recommendation is to consume three servings of vegetables plus two servings of fruit a day. Discuss the use of multivitamins with your healthcare provider. Based on your personal health history, they can make a determination whether you should take a multivitamin.

Vitamins do not promote weight loss, but they can assist in promoting nutritional health.

Food Fit Tips
- Make sure to take your multivitamin with a meal or snack. Fat-soluble vitamins are absorbed with eating.

Do you consume at least three servings of vegetables and two servings of fruit per day?

_____

_____

_____

_____

_____

How often do you currently take a multivitamin?

_____

_____

_____

_____

Based on your health history, what has your doctor recommended regarding multivitamins?

_____

_____

_____

_____

_____

Food Labels

Reading food labels is a part of my everyday life. I don't know if it is the dietitian in me that desires to read them or my desire to be food fit. Depending on your goals, you can analyze the calories, fat, protein, and the carbohydrate content by reading the label.

During both of my weight loss journeys, reading food labels allowed me to watch my total calorie content while enjoying some of my favorite foods.

Food Fit Tips
- Pay close attention to the serving size on each item
- Measure or estimate the amount you plan to consume to ensure you are meeting your goals

How often do you currently read food labels?

_____

_____

_____

_____

_____

If you currently read food labels, what items do you reference on the food label and why?

_____

_____

_____

_____

_____

Day 20

Fad diets

My earliest memories of diets are seeing Slim Fast in my home that my grandma would use. My grandma never ever uttered one word about dieting; however, I knew that she was always trying to watch her weight. I've had so many friends and coworkers that have tried just about every fad diet imaginable.

The truth about fad diets:
1. They restrict calories
2. They often eliminate vital food groups
3. If it doesn't lead to lifelong changes, any weight loss will be temporary.

Food Fit Tips:
- Avoid fad diets
- Eat healthy most often
- Enjoy the foods you love by making the food you choose fit your health goals, your food desires, and your lifestyle.

What fad diets have you tried in the past?

_____
_____
_____
_____
_____

Did it assist you in permanently achieving your weight loss goals?

_____
_____
_____
_____
_____

What are you willing to do now to consistently achieve your food fit goals?

_____
_____
_____
_____
_____

Reflection

You have made it through a whole week of tips so now it is time to reflect.

What habits have you started to change?

_____

_____

_____

_____

_____

What areas can you still improve in?

_____

_____

_____

_____

_____

What are you most proud of this week?

_____

_____

_____

_____

_____

If you struggled in more than two areas, plan how you will do better next week.

_____

_____

_____

_____

_____

If you were successful in implementing three or more healthy habits this week, pat yourself on the back and keep the momentum going.

Food Fit is not a fad, it's your lifestyle.

Emotional Eating

Many of us have been programmed to eat when we are happy, sad, and bored. Think about it. The happiest occasions – such as birthday celebrations, weddings, and absolutely every holiday – typically involve food. During times of sorrow, food is also involved. When someone close to you dies, people bring you and your family food. When the funeral is over, the family goes and eats a meal together.

I am just like everyone else. I too eat when I am happy, sad, and bored. During both of my weight loss journeys, I had to be intentional about watching my emotional eating so that I could meet my weight loss and health goals. Being intentional does not mean that I no longer eat for emotional reasons; however, it means that I am more intentional about my food choices and portion sizes when I am eating emotionally.

Food Fit Tips
- Choose smaller portions and healthier options for the meals/snacks the day before and after a celebration.
- Exercise the day you plan to eat more or plan to enjoy higher-calorie food choices.
- If your emotional eating is due to severe depression, seek the help of a medical professional.

Tasha Sarver

Would you describe yourself as an emotional eater? If so, when are you likely to eat more than normal?

_____
_____
_____
_____
_____

What methods have you tried in the past to decrease your emotional eating?

_____
_____
_____
_____
_____

How do you plan to deal with emotional eating in the future?

_____
_____
_____
_____
_____

Measuring Results

My first attempt at weight loss in my late 20's, I only used the scale to measure my success. I recall getting on the scale every Monday morning. I only weighed in once a week. I was often disappointed when the scale would say the same weight as the previous Monday, or even worse, I would weigh more. I became hesitant at weighing each week because of this method. Even though the scale didn't move much each week, I kept up with my eating and exercise routine. Then one day my friend said to me "you are losing weight." I was so excited that someone noticed my efforts. Soon thereafter, I noticed that my once tight-fitting jeans were so loose that I needed a belt.

As an experienced dietitian at 41 years old, I now know that the best way to measure results is by using several different methods. With my latest weight loss journey, the first thing I noticed when I started to lose weight is that my thighs no longer rubbed together.

Don't let anyone determine what your success looks like. Being Food Fit is all about you. So please yourself.

Food Fit Tips
- Weigh daily & document. Average the weight once a week or once a month for more accurate measurement of loss.
- Measure your chest, waist, hips, buttocks, and thighs once a month to better determine loss of inches (fat loss).
- How do your clothes fit? Do you require a belt? Is your dress too big? Are your underwear too big now?
- Take pictures throughout the process.

How have you measured your results in the past?

_____

_____

_____

_____

_____

How do you plan to measure your results on this Food Fit Journey?

_____

_____

_____

_____

_____

Self-Image

I will be honest. Growing up I had a lot of confidence and I rarely felt poorly about my self-image. I cannot say the same when I was dealing with weight gain in my late 20's and trying to lose weight post-baby. When I am not comfortable with my body weight, my self-image just declines. I don't feel pretty. I'm self-conscious when wearing clothing that reveals my extra weight. I know that many women and men can relate to this. No matter how much my husband says he thinks I'm beautiful, and no matter how much he says he likes my extra curves, I just don't feel good about myself.

I may get down in life, but I never stay there. I used my poor self-image as motivation and drive to become Food Fit once again.

In a society where there are images at every turn of the so-called perfect body, it can be challenging to remember that so many of these images have been airbrushed to look perfect. It can be challenging to remember that some people – both men and women – have had their bodies surgically altered.

Food Fit Tip
- Find images of people who are in your age range that mirror the body image that you aspire to have. Find the images with before and after pictures. Use these images as inspiration, knowing that if they achieved it so can you.

Every social media outlet has people sharing their food and fitness journeys. You can be the next one to share your journey.

How do you see yourself today?

_____

_____

_____

_____

_____

How do you want to see yourself a year from now?

_____

_____

_____

_____

_____

Who are the positive images that you can relate to or look up to?

_____

_____

_____

_____

_____

Support System

I know all too well how difficult it can be to change your lifestyle. We get so comfortable in our day-to-day living that it seems uncomfortable to live any other way. In my first weight loss attempt, I found it very helpful to have a workout partner. It is really easy to cancel a workout only you know about. It takes a lot more effort to cancel when you know someone will be expecting you. My workout partner was a friend of a friend. She invited me to attend an African dance aerobics class twice a week.

My current support system is my husband. He doesn't work out with me and we do not follow the same eating patterns; however, he is aware of my physical fitness goals and he encourages me when I'm doing good. He gives friendly reminders when I can do better. When he saw how much I struggled to leave the house to go to the gym, he bought me a treadmill to remove one of my excuses for not working out.

Food Fit Tips
- Consider asking someone to workout with you.
- Consider asking someone to start eating healthier with you.
- Plan to hold yourself accountable.
- Keep a food and fitness journal.
- Each week plan out which days you will exercise and don't miss your appointment.
- Each week plan out how many days you will prepare your meals vs. dine out.
- Online support groups like Spark People or MyFitnessPal

"If you fail to plan, you are planning to fail." ~Benjamin Franklin

Name 1-2 people who you can include as a part of your support system?

_____

_____

_____

_____

_____

If you do not currently have a support system, name 1-2 people you will ask to be a part of your support system?

_____

_____

_____

_____

_____

Progress Proud

Be proud of your progress. You may not lose weight or inches every week, but what you cannot see is how many more years you have added to your life by being Food Fit. This is your life and your progress, so don't let anyone tell you that you are not doing well. I don't believe that people intend to discourage you, but it happens. I've had someone ask me if I was pregnant when I wasn't. I've had someone tell me I'm too skinny when I wasn't even close to my goal. I always have to remind myself that I have set goals to fit my nutritional health and not someone's perception of what I should look like. When I was overweight, and my thighs rubbed together, there were many people that thought I looked good, but I didn't feel good. I was frequently tired and walking up a flight of stairs was a huge task. No one knows what you really look like unless they have seen you naked. The remarkable thing about clothes is that you can find clothes that fit you well and hide your imperfections. No one knew that when they called me skinny that my stomach would touch my thighs when I sat down. Extra weight in the abdominal area is not good for anyone. Increased abdominal fat can increase your risk for diabetes and heart disease, to name a few.

Food Fit Tips
- Be proud of your progress, it is a journey.
- Kindly ignore people who do not align with your goals for progress.
- Be careful of whose opinion you ask for.

What areas of progress are you proud of?

_____

_____

_____

_____

_____

If you are not progress proud, what are your plans to improve
your progress?

_____

_____

_____

_____

_____

Food Fit Lifestyle

I am, and I have always been a foodie. I love good food. Knowing this about myself, I realize that healthy eating and exercise must be a part of who I am. Otherwise, I will spend my life gaining and losing weight every year. I have found what it takes for me to make my food choices fit my lifestyle and my health goals. I don't believe in diets because they do not last for long. I believe in changing your lifestyle. My goal for this book has been to encourage you to make slight changes each week that will lead to a lifestyle change.

Food Fit Tips
- Find a way of living that involves healthy eating and consistent exercise that fits your food desires, life goals, and health and wellness goals.
- Seek the help of a nutrition professional if necessary. Your health is worth it.
- Be knowledgeable about what works for you.

How have you made Food Fit your lifestyle?

_____

_____

_____

_____

_____

What resources do you need to continue this Food Fit Journey?

_____

_____

_____

_____

Day 28

Reflection

You have made it through four weeks of tips, so now it is time to reflect.

What habits have you changed?

_____

_____

_____

_____

What areas can you still improve in?

_____

_____

_____

_____

What are you most proud of this month?

_____

_____

_____

_____

If you struggled in more than two areas this week, plan how you will do better next week.

_____

_____

_____

_____

If you were successful in implementing three or more healthy habits this week, pat yourself on the back and keep the momentum going.

Your Food Fit Journey has just begun. Focus on making your food choices, fit your health goals, food desires, and your lifestyle.

Made in the USA
Columbia, SC
07 August 2018